MINDFUL HEALING

Positive Affirmations to Promote Health

Robyn Brook and Marsha Brook, M.S.

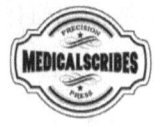

MINDFUL HEALING:
POSITIVE AFFIRMATIONS TO PROMOTE HEALTH
© 2015 Robyn Brook and Marsha Brook, M.S.

Third Edition

ISBN: 1511695889
ISBN-13: 978-1511695886

MEDICAL SCRIBES PRESS. LOS ANGELES, CALIFORNIA

Believe that life is worth living and your belief will create the fact. Be not afraid to live.

—William James

CONTENTS

INTRODUCTION

Affirmations are a tool, a positive declaration the subconscious mind acts on as if it were already true.

When we change our world through positive thoughts, we energize our experiences—even the most challenging—toward creating a healthier reality. This process of repeatedly saying, reading or thinking a positive phrase eliminates the negative self-talk that may have quietly taken hold in our daily thoughts. Through constant daily use, affirmations lay down new roadmaps that direct the brain's subconscious effort toward health and renewal.

Repeating positive phrases (out loud or to yourself) is a powerful way of enlisting your brain in the effort to achieve your health goals. When we affirm things in a positive way, our subconscious mind goes to work, manifesting what we tell it to be true. It is suggested that the mind can best hold about seven words within a thought. We want to integrate these thoughts successfully with visualizations and positive emotions.

YOUR BRAIN IS KEY

Mindfulness and positive affirmations develop that part of your brain which causes the body to calm and heal. In fact, the most current understanding of brain function tells us that *at any age*, new connections can be developed, activating real physical changes in the rest of the body. This brain "plasticity" is key to your healing!

In a complicated system developed over the course of human evolution, the biological machinery of body and mind has developed the ability to activate very real physical changes in the body. The myriad of connections between organs and brain are exquisitely designed to respond to the external environment and our own internal environment as we work to produce balance (or, homeostasis) for survival.

Emotions are part of that system, balancing pleasure and pain, reward and punishment, approach or withdrawal. Change in the body is often initiated by an emotion. Beginning deep within the brain, what first causes us to feel joyful, fearful or sad creates a cascade of bodily responses. All of this activity is transferred from chemical energy to electrical energy and back again.

One way to achieve and integrate new and healthy responses in the brain is the repetition of positive affirmations and visualizations. Using these tools, we condition and train our brains to create a positive circuit of activity between mind and body. While it is a complicated process biologically, the new brain activity sets off electrical guideposts for positive reinforcement.

RELAXATION OF THE BODY

In learning to relax through direct commands, you are truly directing your emotional response system to work in your favor, creating a new and positive emotional state for body, mind and spirit. The associations of different thoughts can cause the secretion of hormones and chemicals in the brain (e.g. oxytocin, endorphins, neurotransmitters and cortisol) ultimately increasing or decreasing the sense of pleasantness you feel.

When we make a conscious effort to relax, specialized routes for pain and healing of tissues can be stimulated too, allowing electrical signals to travel through nerves in the body to locations of pain or distress.

Look to the next section of this book for 4 simple exercises you can use to relax your body and mind.

MINDFULNESS

Take this time of physical rest to allow your mind to rest as well. The practice of "mindfulness" is one where you are learning to be aware of nothing more than the present moment. Mindfulness gives rest to pain and negativity. It isn't magic, but it is magical in it's power for self-renewal. How do you practice mindfulness? Simply listen to each breath. Ignore other sounds around you. Allow any thoughts you have to just float away, always coming back to listening to each breath. Do this for as long as you can. This settling of the mind makes the brain more available for positive direction. Practicing mindfulness before doing your affirmations creates benefits for the brain similar to physical exercise.

Over time, consistent use of the affirmations in this book will bring new awareness. You will be challenged by reality. Your expanded awareness will test this new approach, as daily experiences call upon your new-found positivity. Be assured that as you reassert your affirmations, negativity will slip away. You may even want to add to your affirmations with your own positive realizations.

ACCEPTANCE

When you read affirmations you are nurturing the mind, directing you to feel safe, loved and strengthened, all in the service of increased acceptance. Acceptance is the energizing foundation, the springboard to clarity of thought so necessary to decision-making. Acceptance is where you begin to take responsibility for the direction of your health care. Acceptance is where you will gain insight into the well-meaning efforts of loved ones and your health care team. And it is acceptance that makes it possible to ask for what you need.

You have the power of self-determination. You can listen to the best thinking of those who care and to your own thoughts, and then proceed to make health care decisions that are right for you. Through healthy affirmations, you strengthen your own resolve. Affirmations will help to put you on the right road to reach your healthy goals.

It isn't magic. It is proven that the subconscious mind accepts your thoughts and statements as a given reality. You think one thought at a time and ingest that truth, with the mind seeing your goal as already complete. By giving a positive spin to your thoughts, you give energy to your own inspired goals.

RELAXATION EXERCISES

Using the exercises on the following pages, you can create a peaceful suspension of fear and negativity for yourself. Be patient as you practice these relaxation and present moment awareness techniques.

While these exercises are not required to make your affirmations effective, they can deepen and enhance the experience. Allow your mind to focus and not wander, be open and present, and ready to integrate these powerful healing affirmations as you repeat them.

1

STILLNESS

1. Begin by lying comfortably still.

2. Take a deep breath and move your attention to your toes.

3. Tell the muscles in your toes to *relax*, to go *loose* and *limp*. You are in control.

4. Next, taking deep, calming breaths, move slowly to your feet and send that same message—*relax, loose, limp*.

5. Taking your time, do the same for your ankles, calves, legs and abdomen. And then again—*relax, loose, limp*—for fingers, wrists, elbows and shoulders, neck, face and scalp.

2

BREATH AWARENESS

Awareness of the breath is one way to be present in the moment, creating peace.

1. Close your eyes.

2. Place your hand on your stomach and feel the rise and fall of the movement.

3. Notice the coolness of the air entering the nostrils and leaving.

4. Notice of the expansion of your rib cage. Open fully to the breath of life.

5. Notice if you are withholding breath during the day. Let go of fear and breathe deeply.

3

OPEN FOCUS

Life is like this practice—our awareness is usually limited, as we see only what we are attending to, right in front of us. This technique is a physical reminder that there is so much more to life than what we consciously acknowledge. It's a great way to expand your awareness and can be practiced anywhere, anytime.

1. Look straight ahead and focus on a fixed object or location.

2. While focusing on the spot ahead of you, become aware of all that surrounds you, taking notice without shifting your focus. What do you see?

3. Using your peripheral vision, notice that your vision is greater than this area alone.

4. Take a deep breath. Let the warm wash of peaceful awareness relax you.

4

OPEN ARMS

This practice brings loving energy to the body. It is useful to do this same exercise with all who come to visit you, as hugs are powerful healing tools.

1. If physically possible, extend your arms out from the sides of your body. Hold them gently, palms up or facing inward towards each other.

2. Allow your eyes to drift closed.

3. Take 3 deep breaths and let your shoulders relax.

4. Imagine a great ball of golden energy before you.

5. Allow your arms to curve as you encircle the ball, slowly bringing your hands together in front of you.

6. Embrace the energy and bring it to your chest, holding it to your heart.

HOW TO USE
YOUR AFFIRMATIONS

1. Relax and calm your body, using a mindfulness practice
    or one of the bodily relaxation technique described above.

2. Choose one of the five healing areas from this book:
    Making Decisions, Communication, Acceptance, Self-
    Care or Setting Goals.

3. Pick an affirmation from that section.

4. Repeat the affirmation 3 times slowly. You may say these
    aloud, quietly to yourself, or in your mind.

5. Visualize yourself actively creating this affirmation's
    outcome. An example might be:

    Affirmation:
    "With determination, I advocate for my own health."

    Visualization:
    *I imagine myself in a room with the doctor, smiling and
    actively talking.*

* Create a routine of taking 5-10 minutes during the day for
these relaxation exercises and affirmations. Repeat as often as
possible.

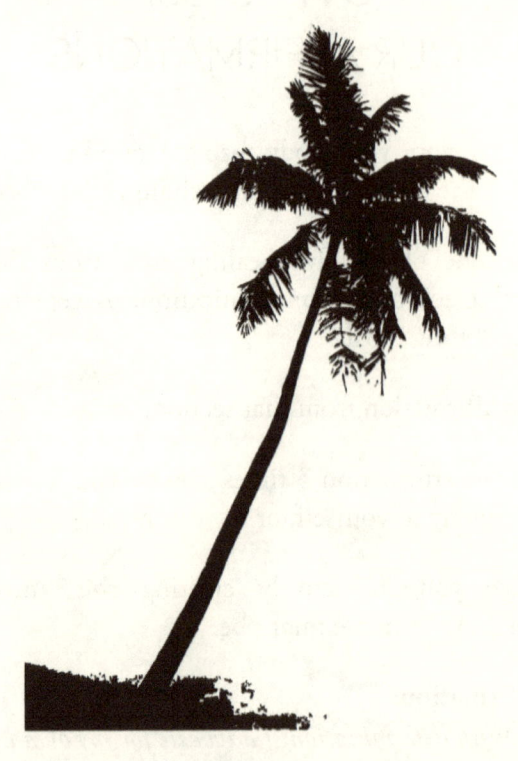

MAKING DECISIONS

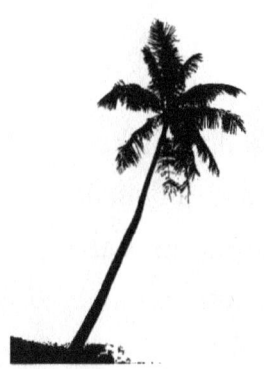

With determination, I advocate for my own health.

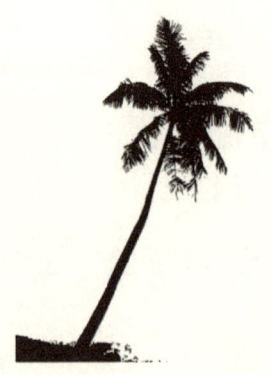

I am empowered to make
decisions based on my beliefs,
and the best thinking of the
community around me.

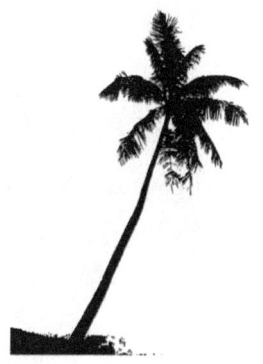

I listen closely to my inner voice, my own source of wisdom. With an open heart, I act upon what I hear.

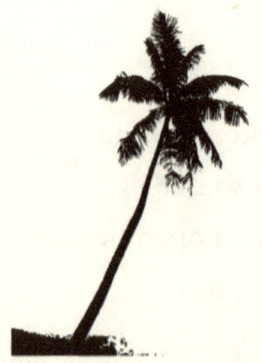

When faced with a choice, I
clear my mind and remain
calm. One thing at a time.

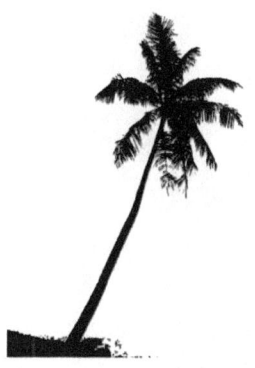

I choose to heal my body with courage and enthusiasm.

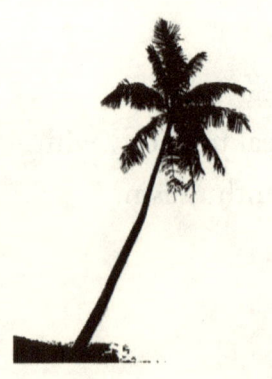

I make efficient use of the energy I have.

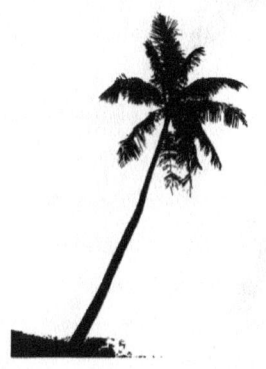

I am a success story.

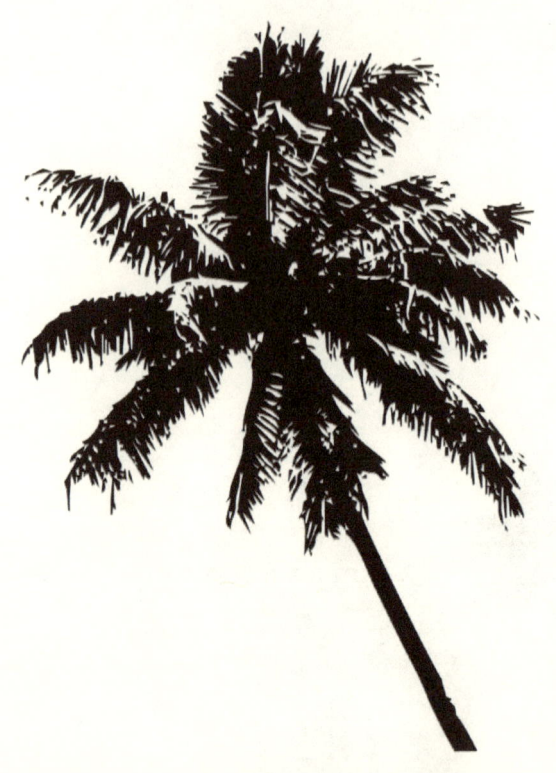

COMMUNICATION

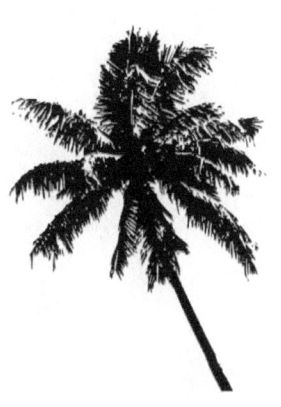

I take responsibility for my health by speaking up for myself with medical professionals.

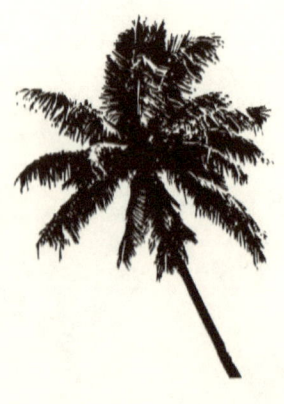

I am courageous. I ask for
what I need for physical
and emotional comfort.

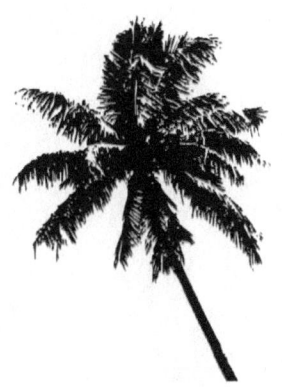

My opinion counts.

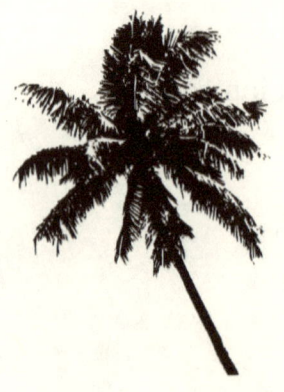

I feel supported by the
wisdom and good
intentions of those
around me.

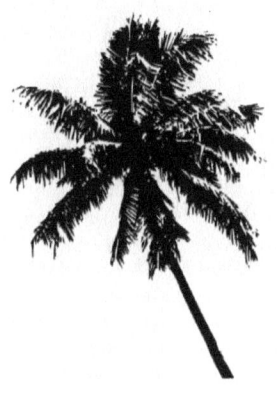

I am my own champion.
I ask for help when I need it.

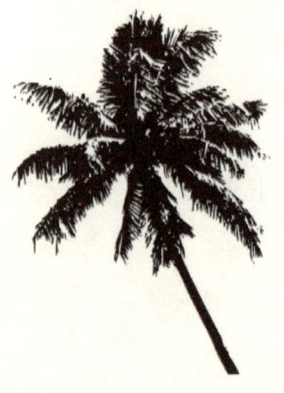

I use the energy I have
for positive thoughts
and actions.

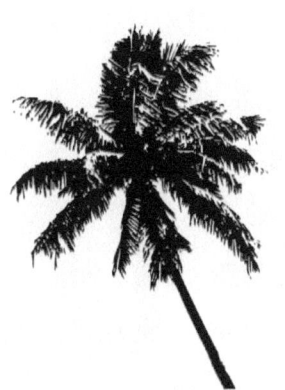

I speak with gratitude to those around me who are here to help.

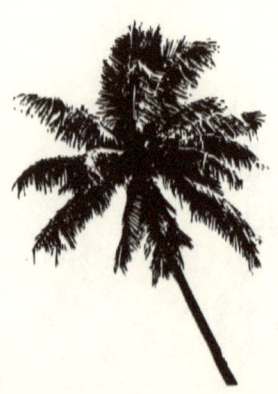

I share in the joy
of others.

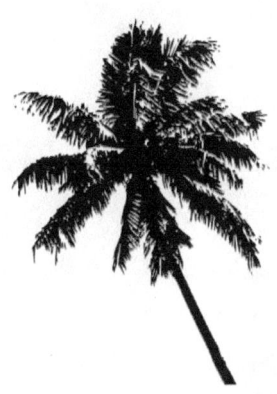

I stay connected to
loving thoughts.

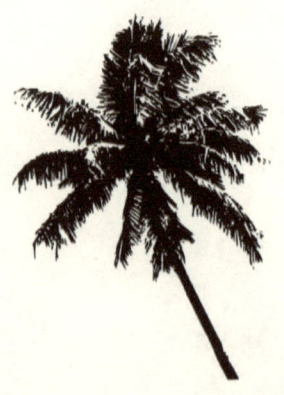

Love surrounds me.
All is well!

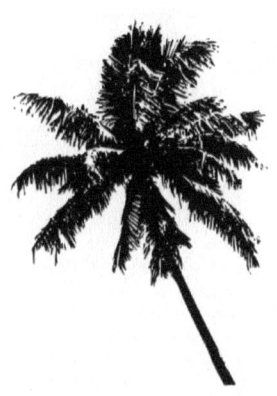

I am my own person.
I create my own story
of renewal.

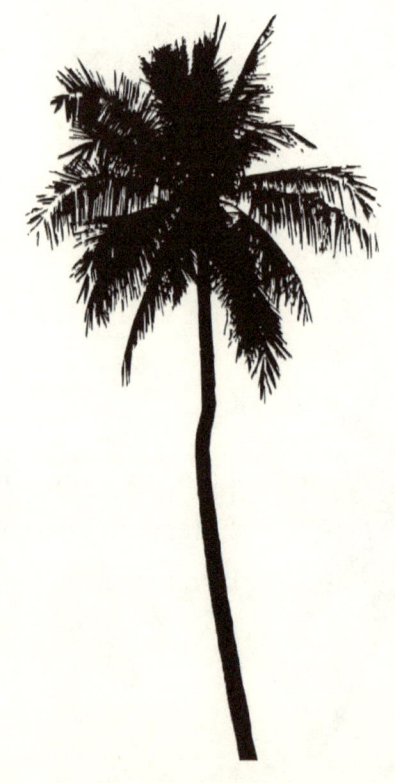

SELF-CARE

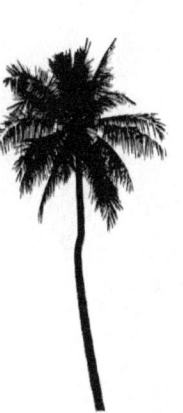

I promise to be gentle with myself
today. I think only good thoughts.

My body is a perfect environment for good health.

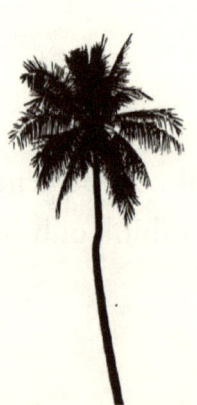

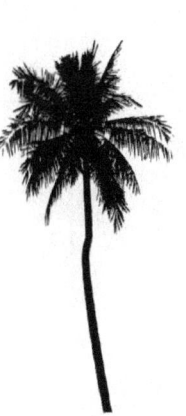

My body is rested
and restored.

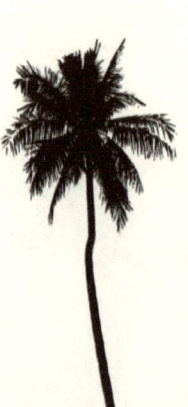

I stay in the moment
to be fully alive.

I am powerful
and resilient.

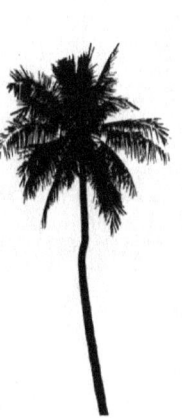

I am fearless. I am motivated
to achieve renewed health.

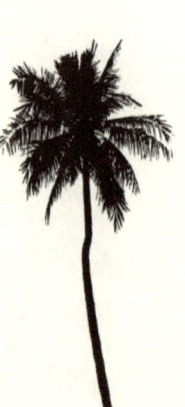

I am my own hero.

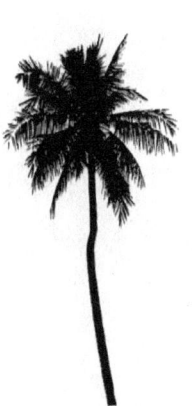

I breathe deeply,
bringing healing oxygen
to every cell of my body.

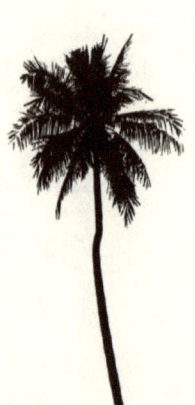

I trust my body.

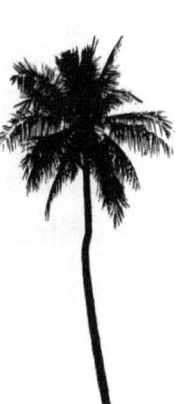

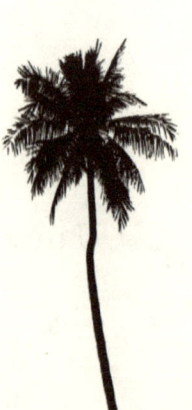

I trust my instincts, even
when I'm feeling emotional.

I say kind and
gentle things to myself.

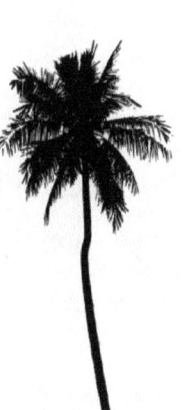

I seek to be positive
in every moment.

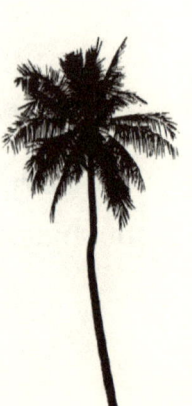

I am doing
the very best that I can.

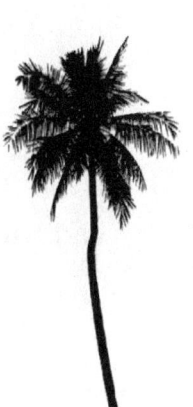

I am truly loved,
and truly blessed.

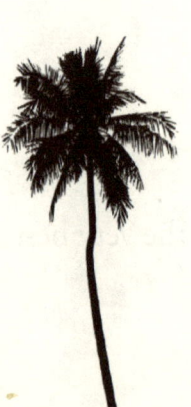

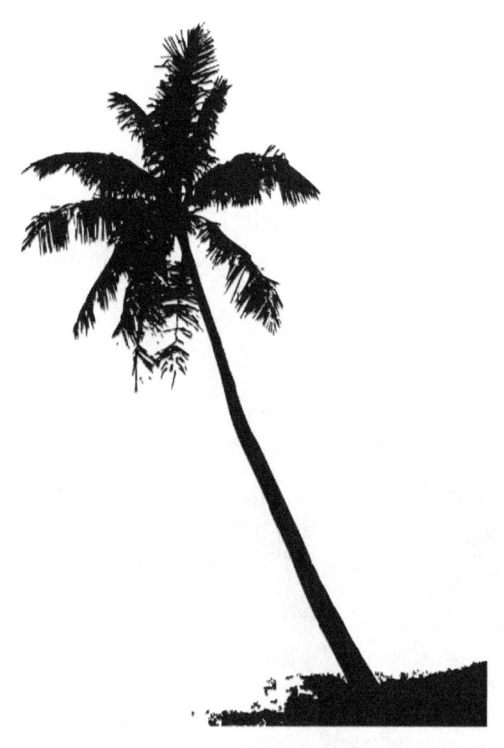

ACCEPTANCE

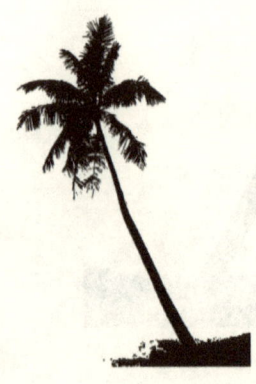

I am ready to accept what is, so
that I can go forward.

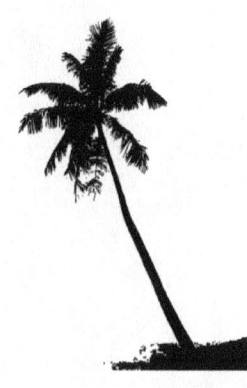

Every day doctors are learning more about my situation. I am in good hands.

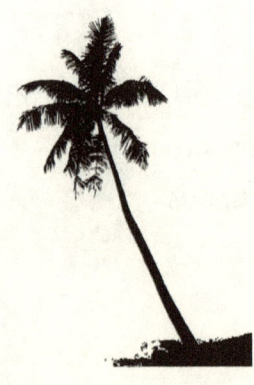

Right now, in this very moment, I am safe.

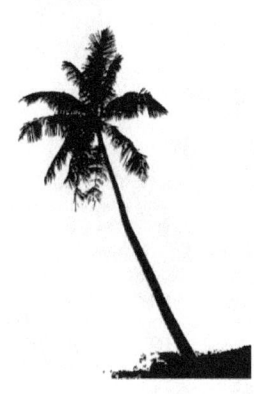

I am truly grateful for this moment, and I free myself from expectations.

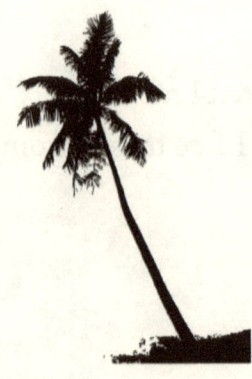

All that is good in life is available to me now.

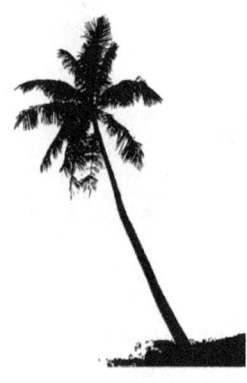

I am grateful for all that
I have today.

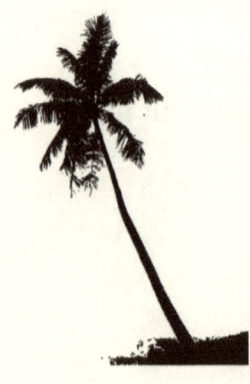

I congratulate myself for all of my efforts, large and small.

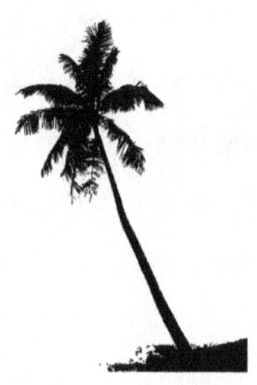

I relax into kindness like a bed of down feathers. I am kind, easily and often.

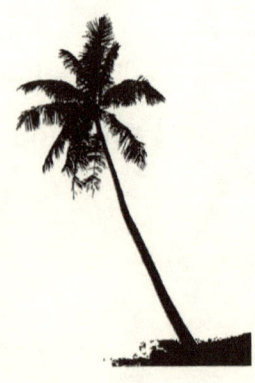

I love to laugh. With laughter comes healing love.

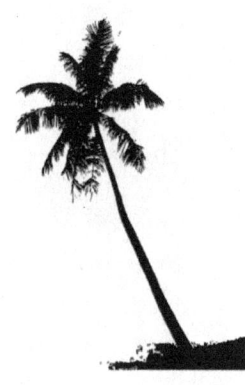

All those around me have
well meant intentions
for my health.

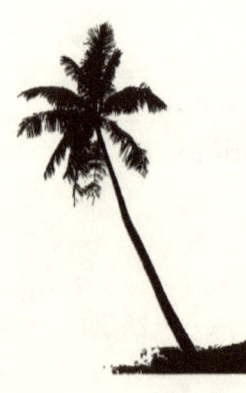

I let go of the "what ifs" in my life. I am engaged in the present moment.

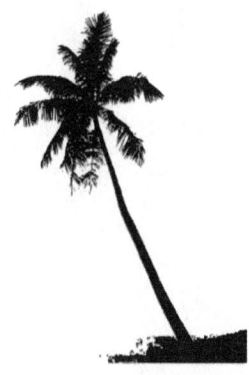

In this moment, I am free and safe from all past hurts.

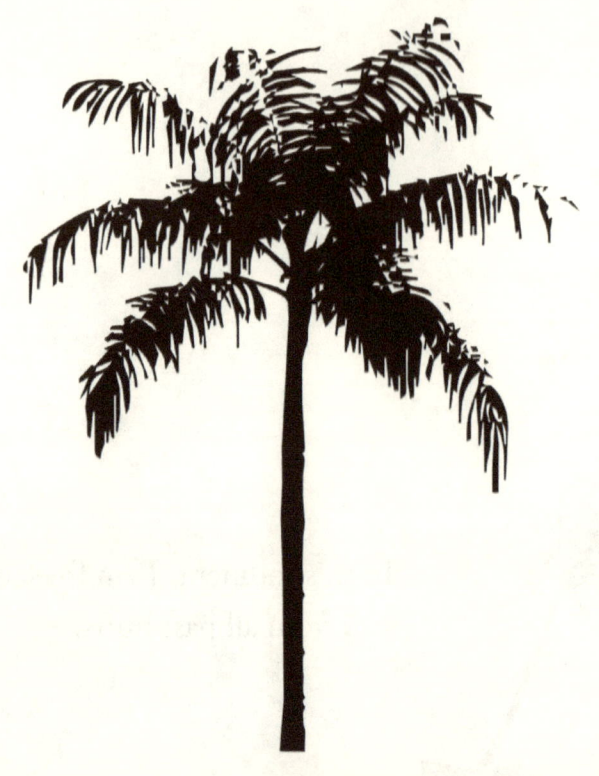

SETTING GOALS

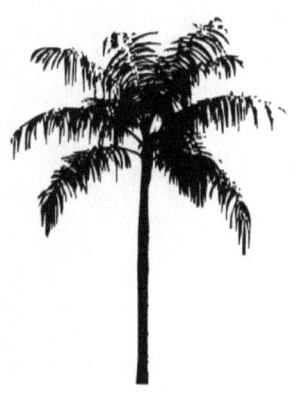

I can think only one
thought at a time, so I
choose to make it
a good one.

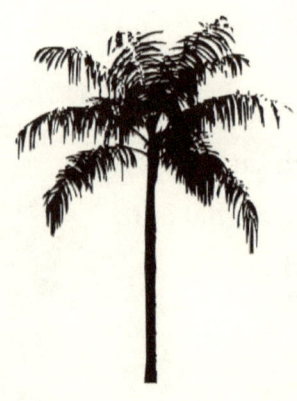

Today only positive
thoughts enter
my mind.

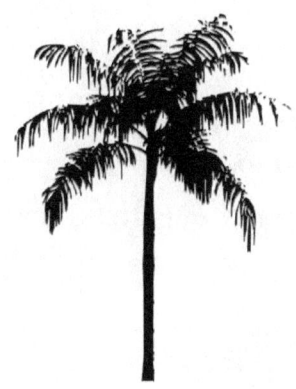

I am progressing toward
abundant health.

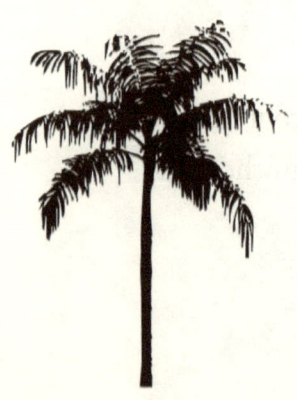

My experiences are steps along the path to perfect health, and I'm grateful for each one.

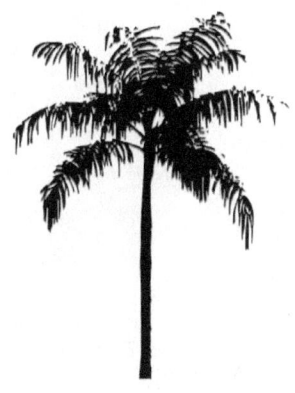

I have the fortitude and
tenacity to accomplish my
goals today.

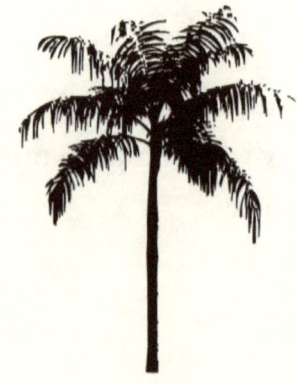

I am focused on success.

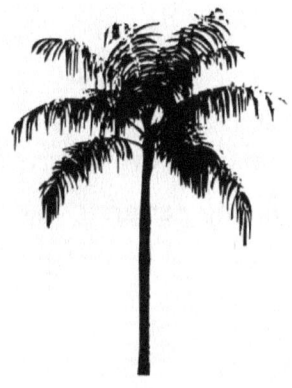 I deserve good health.

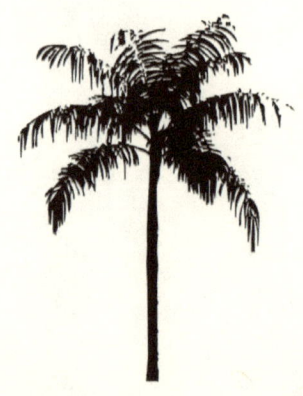

Every day, in every way, I
am getting better.

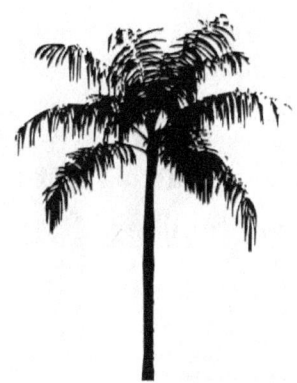

My body is strengthened
through rest.

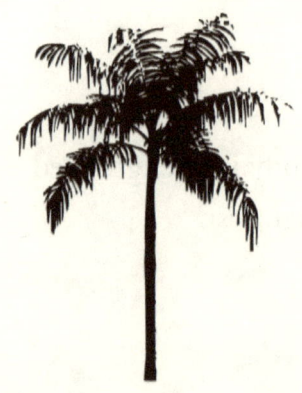

I seek to nurture all that I
am into a fulfilling life.

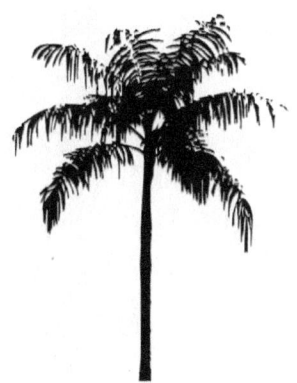

I am restored to abundant good health.

YOUR OWN AFFIRMATIONS

After using these affirmations regularly, you may find that positive words or phrases specific to your situation arise in your mind. Use the blank space on this page to write down the most life-affirming, uplifting ones you discover.

DEDICATION

To Sandy Morrell
& Her Ever-Present Spirit
of Joy, Love and Good Humor

The authors would like to thank the many friends, family and patients who have shared their experience and hope. In so doing, they have helped us to create these affirmations. We offer our heartfelt best wishes for healthy renewal to all who read and use these life-affirming words.

ABOUT THE AUTHORS

Bestselling authors Marsha Brook and Robyn Brook are a mother-daughter writing team. Marsha received her Master's in Nutrition Science from Columbia University. Robyn is a freelance medical writer and bestselling fiction author who received her Bachelor of Arts from McGill University.

For a complete listing of books, excerpts and contests, and to connect with MedicalScribes Press, visit us at:

WWW.MSCRIBESPRESS.COM

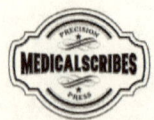

www.ingramcontent.com/pod-product-compliance
Lightning Source LLC
Chambersburg PA
CBHW021413170526
45164CB00002B/627